Myofascial Release

Your Guide to Self-Myofascial Release Techniques with a Tennis Ball

by Merl Buchreich

Table of Contents

Introduction

Myofascial release is an alternative method of alleviating muscle pain and enabling the body to regain its proper mobility and flexibility. This treatment is extremely useful because you can perform the self-myofascial release exercises yourself, in the confines of your own home. More and more people are discovering the benefits of self-healing myofascial release techniques. Its unprecedented popularity is a testament to how effective it is as a therapeutic technique for pain.

With the wide array of pains that people experience today, convenient and do-it-yourself methods are important. If you're experiencing chronic muscle pain and body pains, then you may want to try these self-healing myofascial release techniques at home. Perfectly healthy athletes also love to practice myofascial release to massage their muscles for greater flexibility and to speed up recovery from their strenuous workout routines. It's something that can truly benefit just about anyone.

The exercises presented in this book are simple and easy to follow, not to mention inexpensive yet highly effective. All you'll need is a tennis ball or other similar object. Continue reading to learn more and get started now!

Chapter 1: Understanding Myofascial Release

Myofascial comes from two words "myo," meaning muscles, and "fascial," meaning surrounding areas or connective tissues. These are stretching techniques whose purpose is to reduce chronic body pains to allow you to move around freely.

The Fascia is the elastic material, located between the bones and the skin, which is responsible for protecting the body against foreign organisms. It's also responsible for sending nerve signals about the body's existing condition to the brain. This material is composed of durable, connective tissues that wind themselves around bones, muscles, ligaments, blood and other tissues. It acts like a protective sac that encloses these body structures. By stretching and massaging the fascia in the various parts of the body, several conditions can be eliminated and prevented.

Myofascial release techniques are based on the various trigger points present in your body. These trigger points can cause pain, called referred pain. When the fascia is massaged, endorphins (pain relievers of the body) are released into the bloodstream, lessening pain. The techniques for these exercises involve the use of balls, such as lacrosse, golf, or tennis balls. Rollers are also used as tools for these techniques.

There are myofascial therapists who have undergone specific training for myofascial release. However, if you can't afford one, don't worry; you can easily perform the self-myofascial release exercises at home by yourself. You don't even need to buy expensive equipment.

There are two types of myofascial release treatment:

1. **Direct release**

   In this technique, constant and firm pressure is applied until the release of myofascial restrictions happen. The pressure is stronger than that exerted using the indirect method. You gradually reach deeper into the tight tissues until these are all stretched and the tight spots are released.

2. **Indirect release**

   This utilizes gentle pressure; just enough to relax the tissue. It doesn't dig deep into the tissues. In this method, tissue with the least resistance is targeted.

Is myofascial release treatment for you?

If you've been experiencing chronic pain and no treatment has worked for you, you can try myofascial release treatment (MFRT). There are no life-threatening side effects, so you can adapt the treatment safely. Keep in mind that it's only in trying that you will know whether it is effective.

Are there any preparations for MFRT?

There are no special preparations for the procedure; only that you perform the technique properly. Avoid doing it on a full stomach though, because it will make you uncomfortable.

How often can you perform MFRT?

You can perform it daily for at least 20 minutes. You can increase the frequency and length of time as you get used to the stretching techniques.

Chapter 2:   Self-Healing Myofascial Release Techniques

So, you've decided to adopt these self-healing myofascial release techniques on your own. The first thing that you must keep in mind is that the treatment will not work unless it is done consistently and frequently.

The techniques are simple; all you need for these procedures is a lacrosse, golf, or tennis ball.

To help you with the techniques, here are specific steps you should follow:

WARNING: If you have an existing disease or serious affliction, you should first consult your doctor or an expert therapist before proceeding. It's better to be sure than to be sorry later.

Step #1 – Take a few minutes to relax

Try relaxing for a few minutes. Breathe in and out in slow and deliberate movements. Feel the air move in and out of your lungs. Sit comfortably, with your back straight and your body relaxed. Your muscles can tense up when you start the procedure, but you have to take time to relax for the therapy to succeed. When your muscles are relaxed, you can easily stretch the fascia and gain the results you want.

Step #2 – Identify the painful muscle

Identify what part of your muscles is the most painful. Focus on this area first before proceeding to the less painful areas. If there is no pain, then just search for tight or hard spots in your muscles and loosen them up through myofascial release techniques.

Step #3 – Start with the shoulder

If you have shoulder pain, you can apply pressure to the area using a lacrosse, golf, or tennis ball. You can also use rollers. You do it by placing the ball inside a sock to enable you to hold the ball in place. Hold the end of the sock while performing the procedure.

Stand against a wall, place the ball between your shoulders and the wall by holding the end of the sock, then bend your knees and move your shoulder area against the ball. Position the ball in such a way that it can massage your painful area. You can bend your knees and move your shoulders around to facilitate the stretching.

You can also do this lying down. Choose whatever is most comfortable for you. If you're lying down, you don't need to place the ball inside a sock. Ensure though that the floor is clean, safe and free from any objects that can cause accidents. Place the ball away from the spine and near the shoulder joints. Move your shoulders around to massage the area. Begin with your right shoulder, and then proceed with the left shoulder. Do this for 3 to 5 minutes for each shoulder. The benefit of lying down is that you're using gravity and your own body weight to apply pressure. But if the pressure is too much, start against the wall instead.

Next, place the ball nearer the spine, inside the scapula. Rotate your shoulders to allow the ball to massage the area. If you're using a cylindrical foam roller, you can lie on your side with the roller under your armpit. Your right arm must be above your head. With the roller, start massaging your arm below the shoulder blades. Avoid the armpit area. Do the same with your left arm. Spend 3 to 5 minutes doing this.

Step #4 – Next, address hip pains

If you're experiencing hip pains, you can do this technique lying down. Place the ball between your hip and the floor. Locate the pain and massage the area using the ball by moving your hip around it. Ensure that you don't apply pressure to the area where sciatic nerves are found.

It can be painful at first, so you'll have to use softer balls, but as the massage continues, you'll experience a decrease in your hip pains. The placement of the ball is crucial to the success of this technique; follow the procedures properly.

Step #5 – Proceed to buttock pains

Remain in a lying position. Place the ball under your buttocks. Locate tight muscles and move your body around the ball to massage the tight spots. Roll your buttocks against the ball. You can also move your buttocks in a circular motion to facilitate the massage.

Step #6 – Proceed to general massage

If there are other painful muscles that need a massage, you can work on them first before proceeding to the general massage. General

Myofascial release stretching starts from the shoulders and works downward.

You can perform the shoulder massage as previously described. After the shoulders, you go down the back. Massage the right side first, and then go to the left side. You can also do both simultaneously by moving your body against and around the ball or roller.

Proceed to the muscles of your thighs and legs. Using the same rotating movements, thoroughly massage these areas using a ball or roller. The idea of the technique is to massage the trigger points in the body to relax the muscles, reduce pain and increase mobility.

In cases where pain is absent, there are no strict rules to follow in the order of stretching. So which body part should be treated first? You can either start from the shoulders and work your way down, or start from the feet and work upward. You can also start in the middle portion of your body, should you prefer that method. What's important is that all the muscles in your body are subjected to myofascial release techniques to ensure that treatment is complete.

Chapter 3: Other Variations of Myofascial Release

Practitioners of myofascial release techniques employ a variety of strategies to treat pain. There are various tools available today which can facilitate treatment using myofascial release techniques. Aside from golf and lacrosse balls, rollers are also great options.

<u>Here are some tools you can also adapt:</u>

1. **Grid** - This makes use of a grid-like foam surface that allows various intensities to occur on your muscles through its diverse densities and widths. You can adjust the grid according to your tolerance.

2. **Rumble Roller** - This roller has tiny bumps that can provide more pressure on the muscles in your body. You can control the applied pressure through the tiny bumps.

3. **Quad Roller** - This roller is basically a small rod that has opposite wheels to facilitate the increase of pressure. The wheels make it easy

to maneuver and, therefore, easier to use near joints.

4. **PVC Roller** - This is a tested and reliable roller that you can use anywhere on the body. It's also preferred by other practitioners.

Variations of Myofascial Release Techniques for these different muscles:

A. **Gluteal** – This is composed of 3 muscles of the buttocks: the gluteus maximus, gluteus medius and gluteus minimus. This group of muscles is responsible for maintaining the tone and elasticity of the buttocks.

You can massage these through the following steps:

1. Lean on the right side of your body using your right hand as support.

2. Place the roller under your gluteus muscles. You can cross your knees to feel more comfortable.

3. Let the roller massage your right buttocks from the inside going outwards toward your hip bone. You'll have to move your body to facilitate the motion.

4. Let the roller massage your muscles from the pelvic area going down the thighs. Let your body move to allow the roller to massage the area.

5. Proceed to your left gluteus and do the same procedure.

B. Upper back

You can massage the upper back using the roller with these steps:

1. Lie down with your back on the floor.

2. Bend your knees, placing the soles of your feet flat on the floor.

3. Position the roller under your upper back.

4. Cross both arms across your chest, with each hand holding on to your shoulder blades.

5. Start massaging your back by rolling the roller from the shoulders down to the rib cage's bottom. Roll your back with a 10 degree angle to allow the stretching of your spinal erectors. These are the muscles found along the spine.

6. Do this several times.

C. **Tensor Fasciae Latae** – This is a muscle of the thigh.

You can perform myofascial release massage through the following steps:

1. Lie prone on the floor, with your arms supporting your body.

2. Slightly raise the upper portion of your body.

3. Place the roller under your hip bone.

4. Massage the right portion of your thigh by rolling the roller from your hip bone down to the top of your right thigh.

5. Make sure the other thigh is off the roller and is slightly pointed upward.

6. Massage the right thigh until you feel the tightness disappear.

7. Proceed to the left thigh using the same technique.

8. Do this several times, until you feel the muscle relax and the pain has diminished.

D. Adductors – These are the muscles of the hip.

You can massage these muscles using the following steps:

1. Lie prone on the floor, with your arms supporting your body.

2. The upper portion of your body must be at a 15 degree angle with the floor.

3. Place the roller underneath your thighs. It should be parallel to your body.

4. Raise your right thigh at a 90-degree angle and let it rest on the rollers.

5. Using the rollers, gently stretch your muscles from the hip to the knee.

6. Do this several times, until the tightness of the muscles disappears.

E. Teres Minor – This is a muscle located on the rotator cuff. The rotator cuff is composed of muscles found in the shoulders.

You can massage this muscle using the following steps:

1. Lie down on your side.

2. Raise the right arm above your head.

3. Place the rollers underneath your right arm.

4. Start massaging below the armpit and up to the forearm.

5. Repeat until the muscles relax and the pain has diminished.

You can apply the same technique to other muscles in your body.

Chapter 4: Pros and Cons of Self-Healing Myofascial Release

Just like any other treatment method, there are advantages and disadvantages in performing self-healing myofascial release techniques. Awareness of this will increase your knowledge of the treatment. To better judge if these techniques are the right ones for you, here are the pros and cons:

Pros

1. It's inexpensive – You only need a ball or a roller.

2. You can do it at home – The massage techniques are simple, so you can do it in the comfort of your own home.

3. It's an effective muscle pain therapy – Clinical trials have proven that it works to relieve varied types of pain, such as back pains, generalized muscle pains, and leg and thigh pains.

4. It's safer than medications – Since it's not a drug, there is no chance that it can cause intoxication. Medications have to pass through the liver, where they are metabolized. These are added workloads to the liver.

5. It's easy to do – The steps are simple to perform. Anyone can do it without supervision.

6. Enhances nerve function – Because of the fascia's role in protecting the nerves, nerve function is enhanced.

7. It can improve the quality of life of patients with fibromyalgia – Fibromyalgia is a condition that is characterized by muscle pain, fatigue, headache, joint rigidity and depression. Myofascial release techniques have also eased the pain of persons with fibromyalgia.

8. It boosts the immune system of the body – This is done by promoting the lymphatic system's circulation, thereby protecting the body from infection. Wounds heal faster when the fascia is not damaged.

9. It promotes proper blood circulation – When the fascia is well massaged, the arteries are no longer compressed, promoting proper blood circulation.

10. Improves mobility – Because the fascia's elasticity and consistency is restored through MFRT, joints and muscles will be able to move freely. They're no longer constricted by the fascia.

11. Enhances excretion of metabolic waste – When the circulation is functioning well, the excretion of metabolic waste is enhanced because there are no clogged arteries to stop its excretion.

12. Facilitates entry of nutrients in cells – The faster the blood flows, the easier nutrients reach their intended recipients. Nutrients are needed by the cells in the body, and any delay in their transportation can cause illness or injury.

13. Increases flexibility of muscles and tendons – The muscles and tendons benefit a lot from myofascial release techniques. Because of this,

the range of motion is increased too, and the tight and overly toned muscles are decreased.

14. Aside from easing muscle pains, MFRT also helps in reducing pain in the following conditions:

> Carpal tunnel syndrome
> Plantar fasciitis
> Fibrositis
> Headaches
> Thoracic outlet syndrome

These are some of the conditions with which MFRT can help. Because of its wide range of benefits, MFRT is highly regarded by practitioners as an extraordinary technique.

Cons

1. During the first treatment, it can be painful for sensitive individuals. However, the pain will diminish as the fascia loosens up and greater mobility is restored.

Clearly, there are more pros than cons. MFRT is, therefore, highly recommended for lessening muscle pains due to damage, decreased elasticity and similar conditions.

Chapter 5:   Valuable Tips on Myofascial Release Techniques

To complete your information, here are valuable tips you should observe when performing myofascial release techniques:

1. Applying pressure to your bones will build bone mass. In MFRT, you don't only massage the muscles, but the bones as well. Bones that are not "pressed" will soon deteriorate.

2. It's important to emphasize that "good" pain is expected during initial treatment. Don't stop treatment if you experience pain initially. As long as it is "good" pain – meaning the pain is tolerable and not severe – you can continue with the treatment. You'll get used to it eventually.

3. Use the tool that's best for your body type. Some tools may be too big or too small for your body frame. Choose the massage tool that is suitable for you. This will make your massage more effective. You must also

customize your MFRT based on your muscle pains.

4. Poor posture can contribute to the hardening of the fascia. Hence, maintain your good posture to enhance your fascia's flexibility and integrity.

5. MFRT can be done anytime of the day. There are no restrictions based on time when performing these techniques. Most people prefer it in the morning because it perks up their mobility and motion.

6. For pregnant women, the obstetrician must be consulted first, before using MFRT as a therapeutic method. Depending on the condition of the woman, the stretch therapy may be contraindicated.

7. The ideal tool for the gluteus, calves, shoulders, feet and lower back are balls. Rollers are best for the other parts of the body.

8. The key concept of MFRT is that, for you to be healthy, you should be healthy in mind and body.

9. Anxiety and depression can cause myofascial restrictions. This is because, when you're depressed, your muscles fall and tend to get tight and hard.

10. Elbows and knuckles can also be used as tools for MFRT. If you don't have balls or rollers, you can make use of these. They're equally effective. The problem will be the tiredness of your elbows and knuckles after the massage.

11. When performing MFRT, apply gentle or firm pressure *continuously* to be more effective.

12. One treatment will not be effective. You have to undergo treatment for a certain period of time until the pain subsides.

13. Massage therapy is different from myofascial release techniques. While both use massage as their technique, the focus is different. Massage focuses on the muscle, while MFRT focuses on the fascia, or deep tissue. Massage uses oils, while MFRT doesn't use any liquid.

14. It's essential to treat the whole body. This will prevent the pain from spreading, since the fascia connects to all body parts.

15. Myofascial trigger points can cause sinusitis, headaches and lower back pain. All these can be cured using myofascial release techniques.

Conclusion

Myofascial release techniques are proven to be effective in eliminating chronic muscle pains. Aside from this, there are also several advantages observed among its practitioners. There are still advantages being discovered as the number of people using MFRT has grown. Its many benefits have increased its popularity as an alternative therapeutic technique for a number of muscle and bone conditions.

Myofascial release techniques have obtained a respectable place in healthcare as one of the best alternative methods for muscle pain therapy. With the explosion of technology, MFRT holds a promising future. Discover its awesome effects and benefits by trying the procedure out for yourself.

If you're fed up with medications to cure your pain, then it's time you try this inexpensive, natural technique. It can change the quality of your life forever. There's no harm in trying, so apply the steps that you have learned from this book and improve your health in general. If you haven't tried it yet as you read through the book the first time, give it a try now!

Finally, I'd like to thank you for purchasing this book! If you enjoyed it or found it helpful, I'd greatly appreciate it if you'd take a moment to leave a review on Amazon. Thank you!

Made in United States
North Haven, CT
04 February 2022

15695395R00024